03

10646752

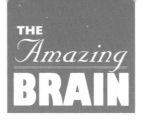

Neurological DISORDERS

By
Connie Goldsmith

Scientific Consultant:
Dr. Paul Thompson
Assistant Professor of Neurology, UCLA

BLACKBIRCH PRESS, INC.

WOODBRIDGE, CONNECTICUT

Published by Blackbirch Press, Inc.
260 Amity Road
Woodbridge, CT 06525
Web site: http://www.blackbirch.com
e-mail: staff@blackbirch.com
© 2001 Blackbirch Press, Inc.

All rights reserved. No part of this book may be reproduced in any form
without permission in writing from Blackbirch Press, Inc., except by a
reviewer.

Printed in Belgium

10 9 8 7 6 5 4 3 2 1

Photo Credits:
Cover, back cover, pages 4, 8, 14, 17–18, 24 (background), 26, 32–33, 35,
40, 42, 55, 56, 59: PhotoDisc; pages 6, 9 (bottom), 10, 20, 28, 36, 47–48,
50, 53, 57: Blackbirch Press, Inc.; pages 9 (top), 16, 22 (top), 27, 30, 39,
41, 44 (bottom): LifeArt; page 11: PhotoSpin; pages 12, 44 (top), 52: Corel
Corporation; page 22 (bottom), 24 (inset): courtesy Centers For Disease
Control, Division of Vector-Borne Infectious Diseases; page 31: courtesy of
Toshiba American Medical Systems, Inc.; page 45: Fox.

Library of Congress Cataloging-in-Publication Data
Goldsmith, Connie, 1945–
     Neurological disorders / by Connie Goldsmith.
         p. cm.—(The amazing brain)
     Includes index.
     ISBN 1-56711-422-9 (hardcover)
     1. Neurology—Juvenile literature. 2. Brain—Diseases—Juvenile
literature. 3. Mental illness—Juvenile literature. [1. Brain. 2. Brain—
Diseases. 3. Brain—Wounds and injuries. 4. Mental illness.] I. Title. II.
Amazing brain series.
RC343 .G564 2001   00-011949
616.8—dc21   CIP
                                                              AC

616.8
GOL
2001

Table of Contents

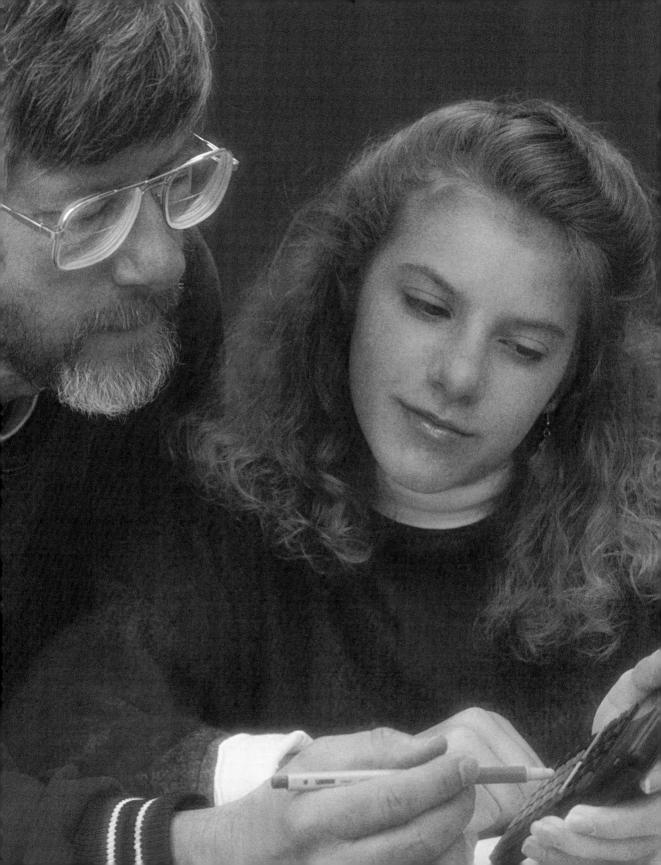

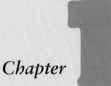

The World's Best Computer

Pain in the Brain

The human brain is the world's best computer, even if it can't add up a million numbers in a nanosecond. Our brains take in a dozen different sensations at the same time, process them, and make a decision in the blink of an eye. A baby reaches out her hand and grabs a stuffed red bear because she likes the color. She looks at its funny face and laughs. A toddler pushes a toy truck through the streets of a pretend city that he constructed from blocks in his living room. Then he decides to take his truck outside and play with it in the sandbox.

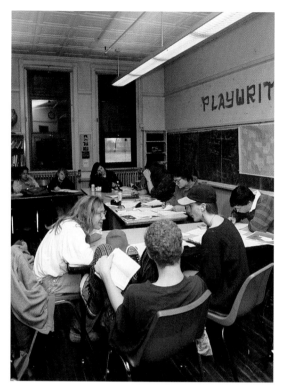

The human brain is able to process input from many different sources at once.

Every day boys and girls sit in classrooms, smelling lunch from the cafeteria kitchen, feeling the hardness of the seats, glancing at trees outside the window, hearing a whisper behind them, thinking about the game on Saturday, deciding what to wear tomorrow, all while taking in new information about math or history. Only the human brain can perform and integrate these complex thinking and sensory activities so effortlessly.

Many things, however, can go wrong with our amazing brain. This book will tell you about some of the neurological disorders that can interrupt the brain's normal work. Some disorders of the brain, such as common headaches, are mostly mild. Other, more serious, brain disorders can be devastating. Neurology—the study of the brain and nerves—is an area of science where new discoveries are constantly made. It's an area of medicine where doctors develop better treatments every day. Neurological disorders that disable or even kill people today may be minor inconveniences tomorrow.

Pain in the Brain

Have you ever had a headache? Have you felt the pounding pain that makes you want to close your eyes and shut out the world? Everyday events like forgetting to do your homework, arguing with your parents, or tripping over your shoelaces can trigger tension headaches. If you sometimes get headaches, you're not alone. Millions of people get headaches, and they often disrupt school and work.

Headaches are the mildest kind of neurological disorder. They're classified as tension headaches (due to muscular contraction), or vascular headaches (due to changes in blood vessels in and around the brain). Most headaches aren't serious, so what causes them and why do they hurt so much? Many things can trigger headaches, such as emotions, fever, foods, allergies, and chemicals. No matter what the trigger, the end result is the same—pain.

Tension Headaches

Special nerve cells called nociceptors (pain receptors) are scattered throughout the human body. When nociceptors are stimulated, they send a message to the brain signaling the presence of pain. If the source of the painful stimulation is in the muscles of the scalp, or in the brain's blood vessels, a headache results. The brain itself can't feel pain because it doesn't have nociceptors.

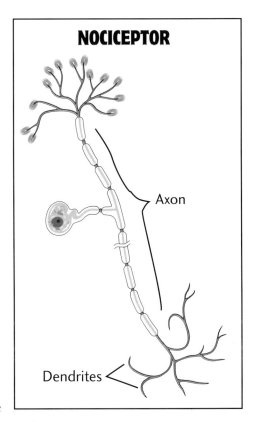

NOCICEPTOR

Axon

Dendrites

Pain receptors, called nociceptors, are special nerve cells that are stimulated by pain.

Nine out of ten headaches are due to tension. Anxiety, stress, and depression can cause painful contractions of muscles in your face, scalp, and neck. The constant pain feels like a tight band around your head. Muscles in the back of your neck clench in painful knots. Even eyestrain can cause headaches.

Vascular Headaches

Blood vessels, which are part of the body's vascular system, contain nociceptors. When blood vessels in and around the brain dilate (expand) or constrict (tighten and get smaller), a vascular headache results. Blood circulation in the brain is affected. Some parts get too much blood, and others don't get enough. The pain of vascular headaches is worse than tension headaches—and

Ancient Cures

Evil spirits inside the skull? A knock on the head by an annoyed ghost? A curse from an angry god? Throughout history, people have tried a lot of weird things to relieve headaches.

Cavemen drilled holes in the skulls of headache sufferers to let out evil spirits causing the pain.

Ancient Sumerians tied a piece of wool into magic knots and wrapped it around the head while praying for relief.

Romans cured headaches by crowning the patient with an herbal wreath.

In 8th-century France, breathing a mixture of vulture brains and oil was believed to cure headaches.

In 9th-century England, headache sufferers drank a mixture of elderberry-seed juice, cow brains, and goat droppings dissolved in vinegar to relieve pain.

Other remedies through the centuries have included flowers, nuts, beetles, belladonna, and beaver testicles!

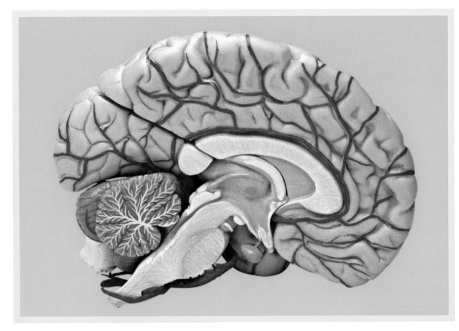

Left: Blood vessels run throughout the brain. When they dilate or constrict abnormally, a vascular headache results. Below: Stress and tension will often trigger a headache.

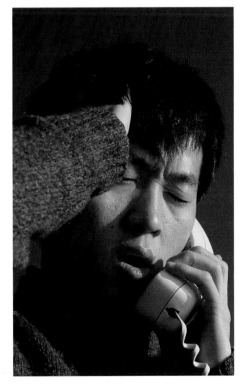

more difficult to manage. A vascular headache often causes throbbing and pulsing, and worsens with activity or moving your head.

Migraine headaches are the most common chronic vascular headaches. They often begin in childhood or adolescence, and are more common in females than males. Migraines are probably tied somewhat to heredity; over half of all migraine sufferers have a family history of migraines.

At the beginning of a migraine, blood vessels constrict, decreasing blood flow to the brain. Some people get neurological symptoms called an aura that can include flashing lights, trouble with speech, or confusion. Then the blood vessels dilate, sending an increased flow of blood to the brain. The stimulation of nociceptors in the brain's blood vessels causes intense pain.

Once the pain begins, it can get so bad that it sends the sufferer to bed in a dark room for hours. Nausea and vomiting often accompany the pain. Migraines can strike people as often as several times a week, or as rarely as every few years.

Most people learn through trial and error what triggers their migraines, and it can be different for everyone. For some, it's stress and tension. For others, it can be fatigue, changing weather, or even certain foods, such as yogurt and nuts, which contain the chemical tyramine. Hormonal changes of menstruation and pregnancy can worsen migraines in women. Prescription medications are often needed to control the pain so people with migraines can live a normal life.

Toxic headaches are another kind of vascular headache. These are caused by fever-producing illnesses or the presence of foreign substances in the body. Some of the chemical culprits that can cause these headaches are nitrites (found in hot dogs, bacon, and lunch meats), monosodium glutamate (MSG—a chemical used to enhance flavors), and even common household pesticides. The goal for treating toxic headaches is to figure out the substance that triggers them and then eliminate it.

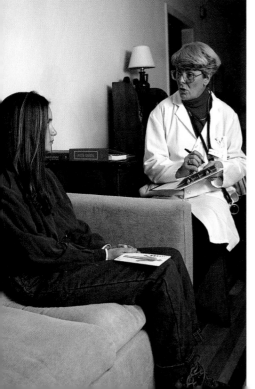

A doctor can help to identify the exact causes of migraines, toxic headaches, or other problems.

Help Me, Doctor!

Most people will never need to see a doctor about their headaches. However, some headaches signal a serious problem (for example, encephalitis or meningitis) that requires medical attention. Talk to a doctor if you experience:

- sudden, severe headaches
- headaches associated with high fever, seizures, or confusion
- headaches after a head injury or a loss of consciousness
- persistent or recurring headaches
- headaches interfering with normal life

Modern Medicines

Most headaches are relieved by common medications that are available without a prescription. Chemical reactions in the body produce substances called prostaglandins that stimulate nociceptors to feel pain. Medications like the ones listed below work by reducing prostaglandins so the brain perceives less pain.

Medication	Side Effects:
Aspirin 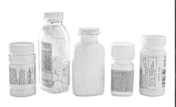	Can cause allergic reactions, ulcers and bleeding from the stomach or intestines. Thins the blood, so excessive bleeding from injuries may occur. Aspirin has been linked to Reye's Syndrome, a rare but serious disease. Many doctors advise against aspirin for anyone under age 16.
Ibuprofen is chemically related to aspirin (brand names Advil, Motrin, Nuprin)	Can cause allergic reactions, skin rash, stomach irritation, and bleeding from stomach or intestines.
Acetaminophen is a good substitute for aspirin and ibuprofen (Tylenol and many other brand names)	Less irritating to the stomach, yet just as good at relieving headaches. However, too much can damage the liver.

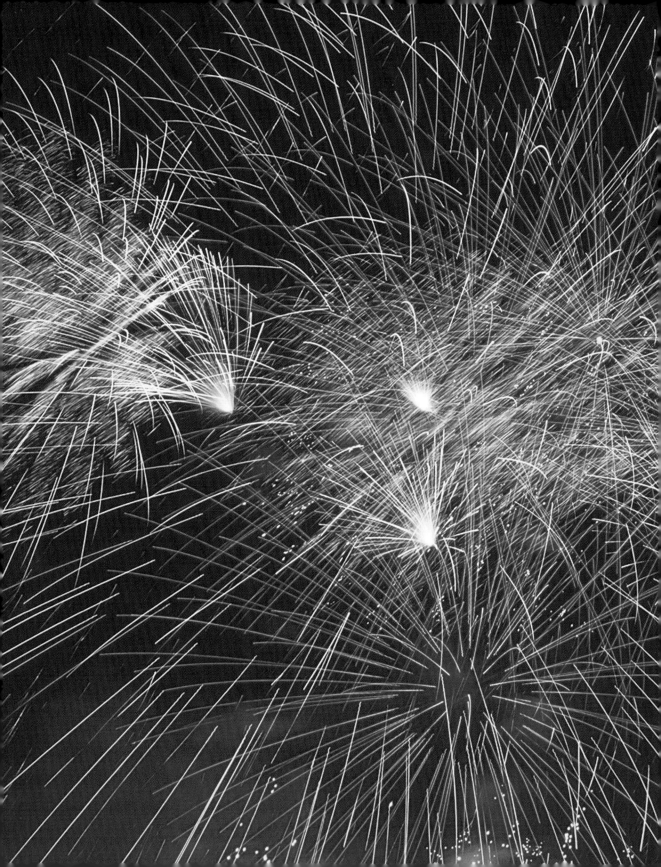

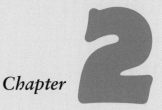

The Injured Brain

Epilepsy and Cerebral Palsy

You've probably seen a Fourth of July fireworks show. Think about a single large rocket going off. It shoots into the dark night sky and bursts into millions of particles that slowly drift down. That's one way to think of a set of nerve impulses going off in the brain. Now think about a fireworks display where dozens of different fireworks are shot off at the same time, different colors, big booms, noisy flashes of light. If each one of those were a set of nerve impulses, that's like epilepsy. The fireworks are beautiful and exciting to look at, but would you want that to happen inside your brain?

In a normal brain, millions of tiny electrical charges pass from the neurons (nerve cells) to all parts of the body in an orderly fashion. When cells in the brain suddenly start firing off at a rapid and irregular rate, a seizure happens. You can think of a seizure like a huge fireworks display, or an electrical storm in the brain.

The term "seizure disorder" is often used instead of epilepsy. You may know someone who has seizures. About 2.5 million people in the United States alone have epilepsy. It is a disorder that often first appears in early childhood. One out of five people with epilepsy develops it by age 5, and half of all sufferers get it by age 25.

Although doctors know many things that can cause epilepsy, in about half of all cases, no specific cause is ever identified. In some cases, a premature or difficult birth can be the cause; in others, genetics or infections may be the reason. Other times, seizure activity can be traced to fevers (especially with babies and young children), brain tumors, strokes, and trauma. Chemical imbalances, such as lead poisoning, low blood sugar, and withdrawal from drugs or alcohol can also trigger seizures.

The type of seizure a person experiences depends on which part of the brain is having the abnormal electrical activity. For example, if neurons start firing

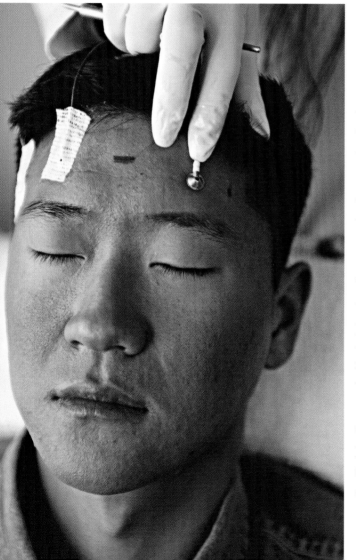

Doctors can monitor brain activity during some seizures to focus on possible causes and cures.

Be a Hero!

If you're with someone who has a seizure, know what to do:

- Call for help.
- Be sure the person is lying flat on the ground or floor.
- Remove any surrounding objects that could cause injury.
- Use a pillow to protect the head.

- Roll the person to one side to keep the tongue from blocking breathing and to prevent saliva from being inhaled.
- Don't force anything into the mouth.
- Don't hold arms and legs down.
- When the seizure is over, the person will be confused or groggy. Protect privacy and dignity until help arrives.

irregularly in the part of the brain that controls vision, a person might see flashes of light. Seizures are broadly classified as:

Partial seizures—only one part of the brain is affected.

- Simple partial seizures: One part of the body loses normal function; for example, there can be jerking of a hand that progresses to the entire arm. Smells, flashes of light, or a repetitive motion, like lip-smacking may be present.
- Complex partial seizures: A person may become confused, have hallucinations, or completely lose consciousness.

Generalized seizures—all or most of the brain is affected.

- Absence seizure (petit mal): These usually occur in children only, who lose consciousness for only a few seconds, but dozens of times a day. The eyelids flutter and the child's activity briefly stops. Many children don't even realize they're having absence seizures.

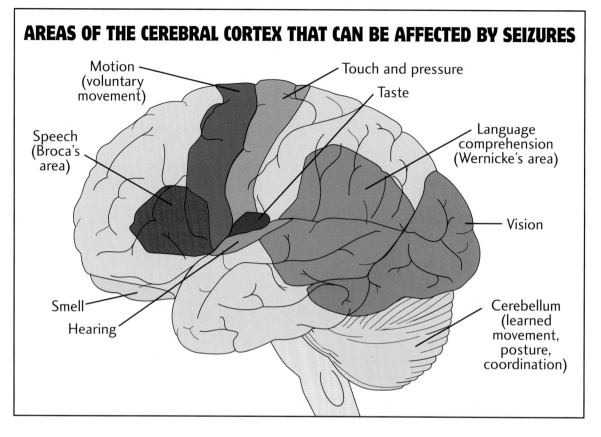

AREAS OF THE CEREBRAL CORTEX THAT CAN BE AFFECTED BY SEIZURES

Motion (voluntary movement)

Touch and pressure

Taste

Speech (Broca's area)

Language comprehension (Wernicke's area)

Vision

Smell

Hearing

Cerebellum (learned movement, posture, coordination)

- Tonic-clonic (grand mal): The person having a tonic-clonic seizure immediately loses consciousness and falls to the ground. Breathing stops and rigidity sets in (tonic phase). Then rhythmic jerking movements begin, lasting for two to three minutes (clonic phase). The person may lose bladder control during the seizure, and will be confused and tired when it's over.

A doctor may suspect epilepsy if someone has a pattern of seizures over time. An electroencephalogram (EEG) helps to confirm the diagnosis. During an EEG, electrodes are placed on the head and connected to a machine that measures the brain's electrical activity.

Dozens of medications are used to help control seizures. Many patients have normal lives with the proper medication.

Seizure Dogs

You've probably seen guide dogs leading their blind owners across the street, helping them to shop, or helping them navigate in a restaurant. You may have seen people in wheelchairs use dogs to open doors or carry things. Did you know that certain dogs help people with seizure disorders?

Roger Reep, Ph.D., associate professor of physiological sciences at the University of Florida, studies "seizure dogs." He focuses on

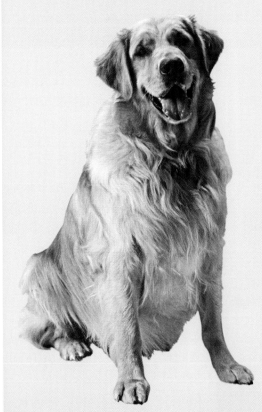

what these special animals can do for people with seizures. Some dogs can alert their owners to an oncoming seizure. Other dogs can help to respond to a seizure already in progress. Dr. Reep says it's important to distinguish between alerting dogs and responding dogs.

Alerting dogs have an uncanny sense of when a family member with epilepsy is about to have a seizure. The dogs may be able to smell a change in the brain's chemistry before the person even knows that a seizure is on the way. The dog barks or whines to warn that a seizure is coming. This gives the person a chance to sit down or get to a safe place before the seizure strikes.

Responding dogs will bark or whine during or after their human owners have seizures. This attention-getting behavior alerts others that help is needed.

Dr. Reep says that no particular breed of dog is best at sensing seizures. Some dogs just seem to be better at it than others. When dogs have that special ability, they can make their owners' lives happier and safer. Some dogs don't require any special training. Others may be trained by organizations that specialize in working with animals for this purpose.

Cerebral Palsy

Imagine this: What if you couldn't stop your leg from moving in circles? What if your right arm was twisted so tightly toward your chest that you couldn't eat or write with it? You might have to go to school in a wheelchair. Your jaw muscles or tongue might be affected. Other kids might not understand what you're trying to say because your speech is slurred. That's what it is like to have cerebral palsy.

Over half a million Americans have cerebral palsy (CP), and about 4,500 babies are diagnosed with it each year. CP is usually identified in infancy or early childhood. Scientists believe CP occurs when areas of the brain that control muscle movements either fail to develop correctly before birth or are damaged during delivery. A brain that is damaged in this way can't control movement or posture correctly. While the exact cause of CP isn't known in most cases, doctors do know some of the situations in which the disease is likely to develop:

Physical therapy can help some people with CP to develop motor skills needed for daily activities.

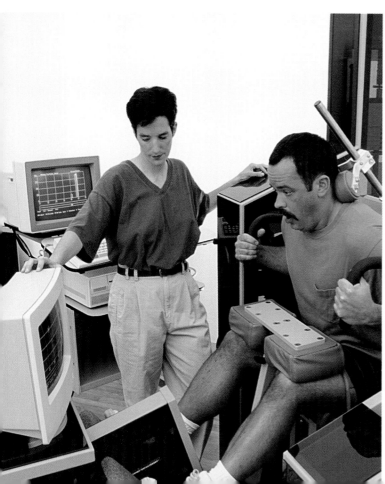

• If a pregnant woman has or gets certain diseases—such as German measles (rubella)—it can interfere with the proper brain development of her fetus.

• Complications during delivery—such as shortage of oxygen or prolonged, difficult delivery—can also cause damage to the brain, which can result in CP.

• Conditions that occur after birth—infections such as meningitis or encephalitis, or a severe brain trauma (bike or car
  accident, fall, abuse)—are other factors that can lead to CP.

Parents of children with CP may notice that their babies don't
crawl or turn over as early as other babies. Some babies will
have muscles that are rigid and stiff. The muscles of others may
be too relaxed, even floppy. Doctors classify CP into four brain-
centered movement disorders:

1. Spastic CP: About 80 percent of CP patients have this type,
   in which muscles are stiff and contracted. If arms are
   affected, writing and eating will be difficult. When legs are
   affected, they may turn in and cross at the knees.
2. Athetoid CP: This type is characterized by uncontrolled,
   slow, twisting movements of hands, arms, or legs. If the face
   is affected, eating or speech problems develop.
3. Ataxic CP: People with this form have poor balance and
   coordination, and tremor may be present in hands or feet.
4. Mixed forms: Some patients have a mix of symptoms, most
   often a combination of spastic and athetoid movements.

CP can also cause other medical problems. While most people
with CP have little or no mental impairment, one-third are
seriously impaired. About half of all children with CP have
seizures. Some have growth problems and suffer from excessive
drooling, poor bladder control, and partial vision or hearing.

Children with CP often get help in a number of ways. Physical
therapy helps to prevent muscle weakness. It also controls
muscle contractures (permanent shortening of muscles) that can
be severely disabling. Occupational therapy is another kind of
therapy for people with CP. This therapy helps to develop the
motor skills needed for daily activities, such as eating and
dressing. For people whose CP has affected the face and neck,
speech therapy helps to develop clear enunciation and word
formation.

SIMMS LIBRARY ALBUQUERQUE ACADEMY

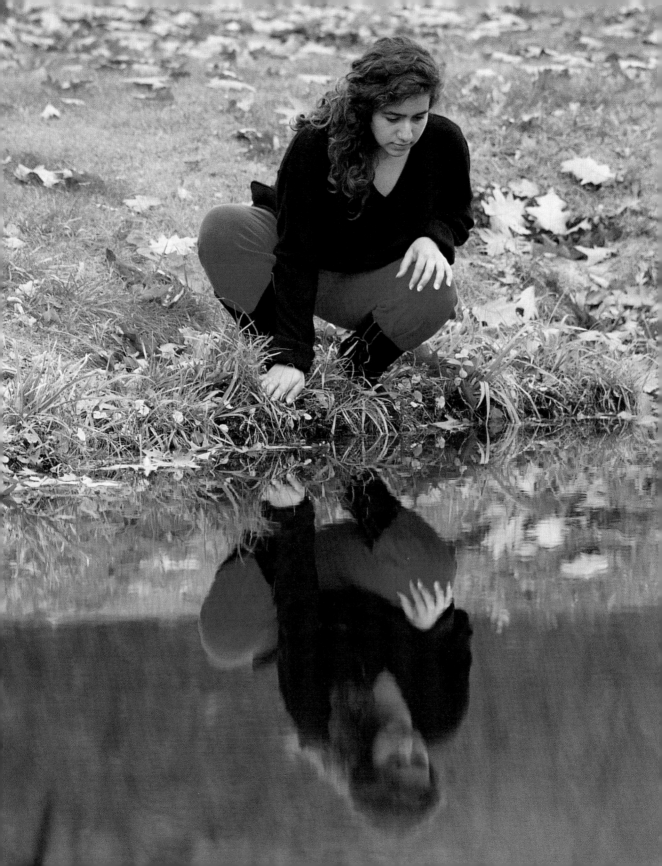

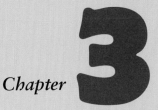

Brain Infections

Lyme Disease, Encephalitis, and Meningitis

You're hiking with your friends on a beautiful spring day. You settle down next to a pond in a big meadow and pull out your lunch. Every once in a while, you feel the sting of a mosquito bite and you flick the annoying insect off your arm. You stretch out in the long grass to rest for 10 minutes before continuing the hike. That evening in the shower, you find a tick in your hair and another on your leg. Don't give it another thought, right?

Wrong! While not every insect that bites you makes you sick, mosquitoes and ticks can infect you with bacteria and viruses. Viruses and bacteria are organisms that can assault your central nervous system (abbreviated as CNS). The CNS is made up of the brain, cranial nerves, and spinal cord. Some CNS infections are mild, but others are serious, even deadly.

THE CENTRAL NERVOUS SYSTEM

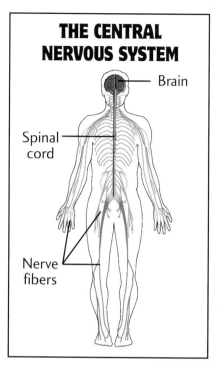

Brain

Spinal cord

Nerve fibers

Lyme Disease

Ticks are arachnids—members of the same family as spiders and mites. They hang on the tips of long grasses, waiting for an animal or person to brush by. When ticks get on you, they search for warm, hairy places where they settle in to feed on your blood. Lyme disease is the most common tick-borne disease in the United States. The bacteria that cause Lyme disease—Borellia burgdorferi—live in the digestive tract of some ticks. When an infected tick bites people or animals, the bite may transmit the disease.

Lyme disease is a potentially serious illness that can affect several parts of the body. Many infected people develop a large, even-edged skin rash around the area of the bite. Others develop a series of even-edged rashes all over their bodies. The rash may feel hot to the touch, but is usually not painful. Lyme rashes vary in size, shape, and color—many have a "bull's eye" appearance—a red spot surrounded by a clear ring, around which is another red circle.

Below: Certain ticks—mostly deer ticks—can carry the bacteria that cause Lyme disease. Below right: Even-edged, red rashes are a common symptom of Lyme disease.

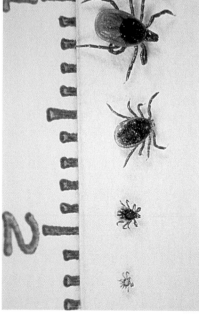

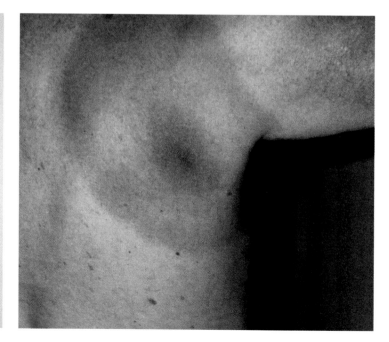

The early stage of Lyme disease feels like the flu, with fever, swollen lymph nodes, and headaches. In the later stages, the bacteria can attack the brain and paralyze muscles of the face, a condition called Bell's palsy. The bacteria can also cause meningitis, which is an infection of the membranes that cover the brain and spinal cord. Lyme disease can also cause arthritis, heart problems, and in rare cases, death.

Doctors will suspect Lyme disease if someone with these symptoms lives in a tick-infested area or remembers being bitten by a tick. A blood test will confirm the diagnosis. If the patient has neurological symptoms, a doctor often performs a spinal tap to obtain a sample of spinal fluid to test for the Lyme disease bacteria. Using a local anesthetic, a needle is inserted between the vertebrae of the lower back into the spinal canal where the spinal fluid circulates, and a sample is taken.

Lyme disease is treated with oral or intravenous antibiotics. Most people have a good recovery, but some have lasting symptoms. A new vaccine for people between the ages of 15 and 70 years old has recently become available. The vaccine can reduce the risk of getting the disease by about 80 percent. It is expected to be approved for younger people soon. Your doctor can tell you if the vaccine is right for you.

Encephalitis

What would you feel like if one of those mosquitoes that bit you on the hike gave you encephalitis? For one thing, you would have a sudden fever and a bad headache. You might vomit or get photophobia (oversensitivity to light). You might become disoriented and confused. You could even have seizures or go into a coma (a deep state of unconsciousness).

The seriousness of encephalitis depends on a person's age, health, and the strain of virus that takes hold in the brain. Symptoms of encephalitis vary from a mild, flu-like illness, to a serious life-threatening condition. Some encephalitis survivors are left with permanent brain damage. Eastern Equine Encephalitis, first identified in the United States in 1930, has a fatality rate as high as 30 percent.

Encephalitis is a sudden inflammation or swelling of the brain, most often due to a virus carried by a mosquito. Encephalitis is dangerous because brain swelling pushes delicate tissue against the inside of the hard skull. Neurons are damaged by increased pressure and by the body's own immune response. The presence of infection triggers the body to send an army of white blood cells to battle the invader. Although the white blood cells are meant to help, they can actually be harmful. The cells can block tiny vessels in the brain, which can cause bleeding.

There isn't a vaccine for encephalitis in humans yet. Most cases of viral encephalitis can't be treated with antibiotics—there are no known drugs that can kill viruses.

Some mosquitoes carry the virus that causes encephalitis in humans. The best way to prevent encephalitis is to control mosquito populations.

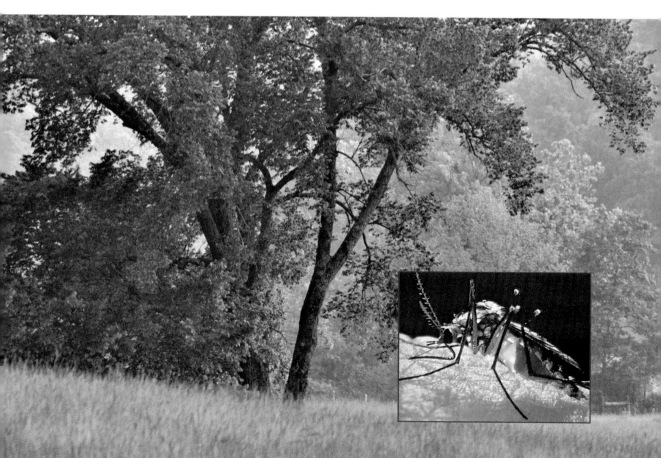

The rise in encephalitis cases in the United States is due to increased mosquito populations. The virus lives in birds and mammals. Mosquitoes feed on the blood of infected animals and can transmit the virus when they bite humans. The best way to prevent encephalitis is to control mosquitoes. In areas with heavy mosquito populations, public health officials may order the use of spray insecticides or other measures to kill these potentially dangerous pests.

Meningitis

Imagine that your neck and back were so stiff and painful that you couldn't even bend them. If this problem were accompanied by a high fever and a severe headache, you might have meningitis. Meningitis is more common than encephalitis, and its symptoms are similar. Neck and back pain, however, signal that the illness is meningitis.

Three layers of tissue-thin membranes—called meninges—help protect and cushion the brain and spinal cord. The cerebrospinal fluid (abbreviated as CSF) circulates between the meninges and brain, adding another layer of protection. Meningitis occurs when bacteria or viruses infect the meninges and CSF.

Common cold and flu viruses sometimes cause mild cases of viral meningitis. These cases last less than ten days and seldom require hospitalization. Bacterial meningitis, however, is very serious. Most cases of bacterial meningitis are caused by the meningococcus, pneumococcus, or Hemophilus influenzae bacteria.

The bacteria are passed from person to person through respiratory secretions released by breathing, sneezing, or contact with mucus. When bacteria reach the meninges, they can damage nerves and blood vessels. The brain continually produces CSF. If its normal flow is blocked by infection, there's a dangerous increase of pressure inside the brain. The bacteria also produce harmful chemical byproducts as they multiply. As is true with

Killer Mosquitoes and Sentinel Chickens

What's eating you? If you're outdoors, chances are it's a mosquito. These blood-sucking pests can be downright dangerous. Mosquitoes carry encephalitis, malaria, and yellow fever. They can even infect your pets with heart worms. In 1999, West Nile encephalitis, a disease never before seen in the United States, broke out in New York City. The culprit? Mosquitoes.

When the smell of blood attracts a mosquito to you, she (it's always a female) injects saliva laced with a blood-thinning anticoagulant into your skin. It's the mosquito's saliva that carries the viruses and bacteria that make people sick.

Mosquitoes breed in water. Even small amounts of stagnant water trapped in a rusty can or an old tire will serve as a mosquito nursery. Dump any standing water that is around your house to help control mosquitoes.

Public health officials use flocks of sentinel chickens to track the spread of encephalitis. When mosquitoes carrying encephalitis bite chickens, the chickens develop antibodies (substances produced to fight invading organisms) to the foreign virus.

The chickens get their blood tested every few weeks. If antibodies for encephalitis are present, officials notify the public about a possible outbreak of the disease. Nearly 20 states now monitor for West Nile encephalitis.

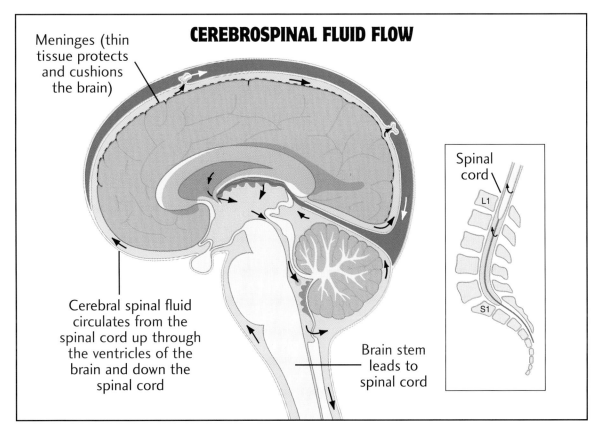

CEREBROSPINAL FLUID FLOW

Meninges (thin tissue protects and cushions the brain)

Spinal cord

L1

S1

Cerebral spinal fluid circulates from the spinal cord up through the ventricles of the brain and down the spinal cord

Brain stem leads to spinal cord

encephalitis, both the invading organism and the body's own immune response to it can cause neurological damage.

People with possible bacterial meningitis must be admitted to a hospital for urgent care. The disease can be lethal in just hours or a day. To check for meningitis, a doctor will do a spinal tap to obtain a sample of the CSF. If the CSF shows bacteria, antibiotics will be started. With early diagnosis and treatment, about 90 percent of patients with bacterial meningitis recover.

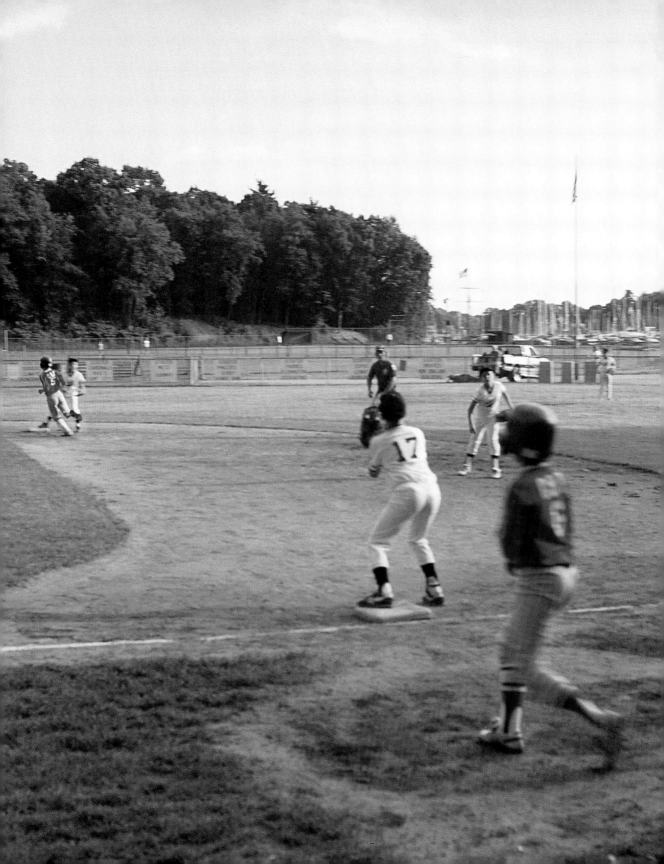

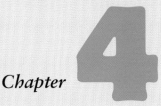

Chapter

Pressure on the Brain

Hydrocephalus, Brain Tumors, and Coma

Did you ever get hit hard by a baseball or bang into something hard? Think of how much it hurt. Remember the swelling and the bruising? Swelling is the body's normal response to injury. The fluid that fills the injured area protects it and begins the healing process. A big purple bruise means blood vessels have broken under your skin. After a few days, as the blood is reabsorbed into the body, a bruise will finally disappear. Swelling and bruising are bad enough when they're on your arm or leg, but inside the brain, they can be deadly.

Brain tissue is very delicate. The three-pound human brain contains billions of neurons and nerve fibers. A hard skull fits tightly over the brain and helps protect it from injury. The skull leaves the brain with little room to expand, so even minor swelling can create dangerous pressure. Various things can cause the brain to swell. Accidents, tumors, and a condition called hydrocephalus are some of the most common conditions that can create dangerous pressure on the brain.

Hydrocephalus

Cerebrospinal fluid (CSF) is created and circulated through spaces in the brain called ventricles. Small canals connect ventricles to each other and to the space around the spinal cord. CSF cushions the brain and spinal cord. It also delivers nutrients to the brain and removes wastes. CSF is normally absorbed into the bloodstream as fast as it is produced. When ventricles or canals are blocked, CSF quickly builds up inside the brain, increasing pressure to dangerous levels.

About 1 out of every 500 children has hydrocephalus. Often, it is detected before birth by routine ultrasounds that are done during pregnancy. Sometimes hydrocephalus isn't found until after birth, or it develops in very early childhood. Because an infant's skull is soft, a baby with hydrocephalus will have a noticeably enlarged head from excessive CSF.

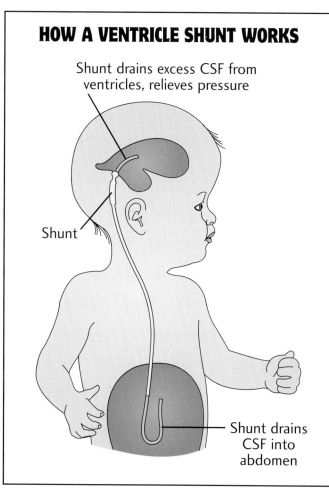

HOW A VENTRICLE SHUNT WORKS

Shunt drains excess CSF from ventricles, relieves pressure

Shunt

Shunt drains CSF into abdomen

When older children or adults get hydrocephalus due to trauma, tumors, strokes, or other reasons, the symptoms are different. The head does not get larger because the skull is hard and its bones have fused. Instead, symptoms include headaches, vomiting, nausea, and problems with vision, balance, and coordination.

When hydrocephalus strikes, it is critical to relieve the pressure on the brain as soon as possible. If there is too much pressure for too long, permanent brain damage occurs. In most cases, a device called a shunt is used to drain excess CSF from the brain. One end of a tube is placed into a ventricle. A surgeon tunnels the tube from the brain under the skin of the neck and down into the abdomen or heart. A one-way valve keeps CSF flowing from the brain out the end of the shunt. Before shunts were invented, hydrocephalus was nearly always fatal. Today, when uncomplicated hydrocephalus is quickly treated, most children will lead normal lives.

MRI and CT scans (like the image below) help doctors to get a clear picture of what is inside the brain. Here, lower left, a tumor can be seen.

Brain Tumors

A tumor is an abnormally rapid growth of tissue, or a form of cancer. Brain tumors can be as small as a pea or as large as an egg. Some brain tumors are benign, which means they will probably not spread to other parts of the body, and, once removed, will probably not return. Other tumors are malignant, which means that metastasis (spreading to other parts of the body) is likely. It can be very difficult to completely rid the body of a malignant tumor. Cancerous brain cells can get into the brain in various ways. Their

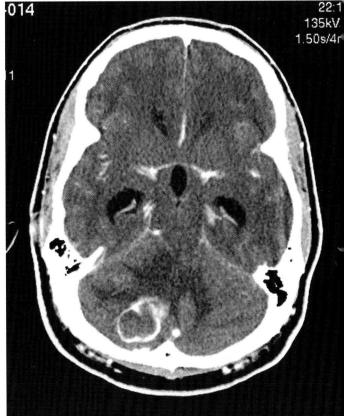

growth can begin inside the brain. They can also travel to the brain from other parts of the body, such as lungs and breasts. Whether the tumor is benign or malignant, as it grows, it puts pressure on the brain.

About 40,000 people a year get brain tumors, and they can happen at any age. When children get them, it is often between ages 6 and 9. However, most brain tumors occur in older people. Symptoms of brain tumors depend on where in the brain the tumor is growing. As a tumor puts increased pressure on brain tissue, symptoms can include:

- headaches
- seizures
- nausea and vomiting
- problems with seeing or hearing
- problems with balance and motion
- problems with thinking, memory, and behavior

When a doctor suspects a brain tumor, special tests called CT and MRI scans are done. These show doctors what is going on inside the brain. A surgeon might need to drill a small hole in the skull and remove a tiny piece of the tumor in order to examine it under a microscope.

Most people with a brain tumor need an operation to remove as much of it as possible. After the surgeon has drilled through the skull, a microscope is used to see the tumor. The surgeon may cut the tumor out, or may use special laser light beams to destroy it. If a tumor is malignant, the patient may need radiation therapy or chemotherapy. Radiation therapy attacks the tumor with strong X-rays. Chemotherapy attacks with strong tumor-killing drugs.

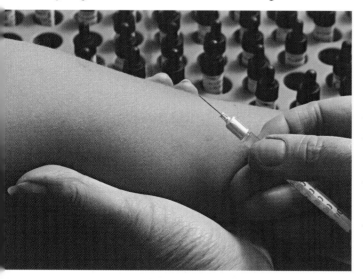

Chemotherapy is one kind of treatment for cancer. Chemotherapy attacks tumors with strong drugs.

Helmets Help!

Traumatic brain injury is the most common cause of disability and death among children and adolescents in the United States.

Each year, more than 1 million young people sustain brain injury, and more than 30,000 of them suffer permanent disability. The vast majority of these injuries could have been lessened or avoided by following these three simple rules:

1. Wear bicycle helmets every time you're on a bike. Bicycle riders without helmets are 14 times more likely to be killed in an accident than are riders with helmets. Helmets decrease the risk of serious head injury by 85 percent.

2. If you use a motorcycle, always wear a motor-cycle helmet, whether you're a passenger or the driver.

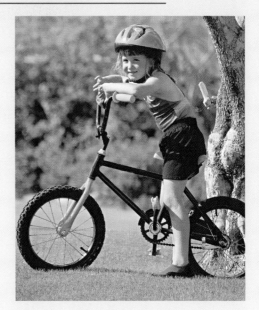

3. Always wear seat belts in a car, and be sure children sit in proper child safety seats. Never put young children in the front seat of a car with air bags.

If a brain tumor is benign, a person can have a full recovery if the pressure on the brain is relieved quickly. People with malignant tumors may have a partial recovery if most of the tumor is removed. Sometimes tumors grow back. Scientists are working to find better ways to diagnose and treat all kinds of brain tumors.

Coma and Brain Death

In the movies and on television, people wake up from comas all the time. In real life, however, it isn't that simple. People in comas are in a deep state of unconsciousness. They can't think, talk, or respond to other people. They can't tell you if something hurts or if they are hungry. If their bodies move, it is involuntary (uncontrolled and unintentional). A coma happens when there is damage to parts of the brain that control awareness, thought, speech, and movement. Because brain tissue is so fragile, many different things can cause a coma:

Chemical-related causes:

- Overdoses of certain drugs, such as prescription sleeping pills and pain medications, can bring on a coma. Excessive amounts of narcotics, such as morphine and heroin, can also be causes.
- Very low blood sugar can be the source of a coma. The brain simply cannot function without a continuous supply of glucose (simple sugar) in the blood.

Lack of oxygen to the brain:

- Choking, near drowning, or breathing carbon monoxide rob the brain of much-needed oxygen. Without oxygen, the brain shuts down.
- A stroke that cuts off some of the brain's blood supply can also be a cause of coma. Blood carries oxygen throughout the body, so restricting its flow can create an oxygen deficiency.

Pressure on the brain:

- From trauma, such as an accident or gunshot wound, a burst blood vessel, brain tumors, or hydrocephalus, the buildup of blood in the brain creates dangerous pressure.

Depending on the extent of damage to the brain, a person may or may not wake from a coma. Some people wake up completely normal after a coma. Some wake up with neurological damage, such as problems speaking or weakness on one side. Other people may wake but may remain in what is called a vegetative state. Their eyes may be open, and they may move a little bit, make sounds and seem awake, but someone in a

Mari's Brain Tumor

Mari was 7 years old when she started having severe headaches and blurred vision. When her pediatrician examined her eyes, he noticed symptoms of increased pressure in the brain. Mari had a CT scan that showed a dangerous brain tumor called an astrocytoma growing in her cerebellum. A few days later, Mari began vomiting and having double vision, common symptoms of increasing brain pressure.

She was immediately taken to the hospital where doctors performed surgery to remove the brain tumor. For the next 10 years, Mari had repeat brain scans to be sure the tumor didn't return. When she turned 17, her last brain scan was negative and doctors pronounced her cured.

Organizations such as the National Institute of Neurological Disorders and Stroke, The American Brain Tumor Association, and the National Brain Tumor Foundation sponsor research into the causes and treatments of brain tumors. As new and exciting advances are made each year, patients and doctors look forward to improved therapies for brain tumors.

Some key areas of brain tumor research include:

1. Implanting radioactive pellets and tiny wafers soaked with cancer-fighting drugs directly into the tumor.

2. Using an instrument called a Gamma knife to do surgery without cutting into the head.

3. Hyperthermia, which uses microwaves to destroy tumor cells.

4. Using substances called monoclonal antibodies to specifically target tumor cells and destroy them.

vegetative state has little brain function and cannot react to the environment.

Sometimes damage to the brain is so severe that there is no hope of the person ever regaining consciousness. In these cases, machines are needed to keep the body alive. At this point, a doctor may determine that a person is "brain dead." Several EEGs will show if there is any electrical activity in the brain.

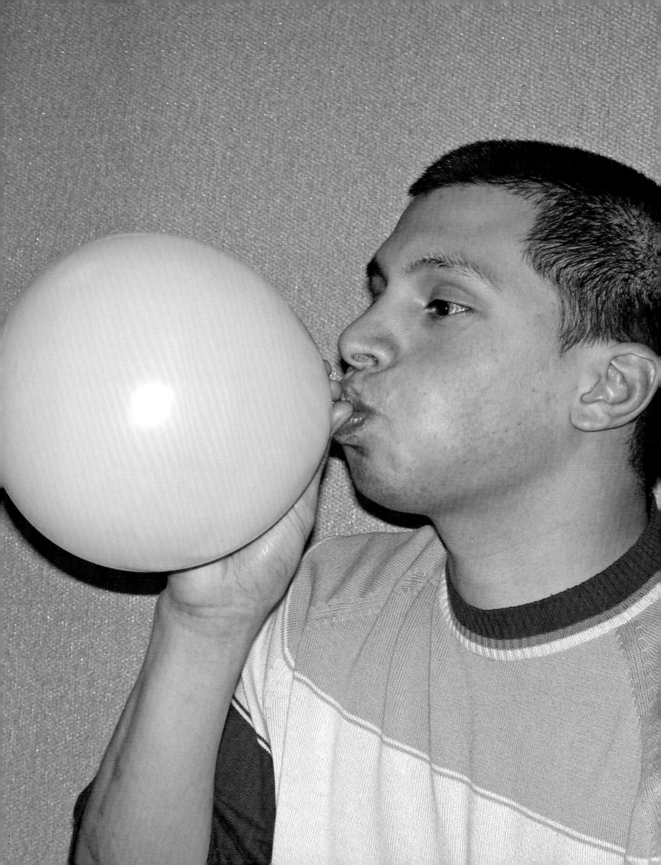

Circulatory Problems

Aneurysm and Stroke

Your brain is the hungriest organ in your body. Even though your three-pound brain is only a tiny fraction of your entire weight, it consumes about one-fifth of your body's energy supplies of oxygen and glucose! Oxygen and glucose are both carried in blood. Anything that interrupts the normal flow of that blood can damage the brain in just a few minutes.

Aneurysm—Blowout in the Brain

Did you ever throw a water balloon and watch it burst on road or sidewalk? Remember the big puddle of water it left? Did you ever blow up a balloon so big that it popped in your face? Did you notice the ragged edges around the hole?

Imagine that one of the blood vessels in your brain has a weak spot. Blood is rushing through the artery or vein. The weak spot begins to swell just like a balloon with too much air or water. When the weak spot builds up too much pressure, the blood vessel ruptures, or explodes. Blood gushes out of the hole into surrounding brain tissue, like the puddle of water left by a broken water balloon.

A brain aneurysm is a weakness in a vessel wall. It can be present at birth, or it can be caused by high blood pressure or trauma. Not all aneurysms burst. Some people may have them their entire lives. When an aneurysm does burst, however, it is a life-threatening emergency. The escaping blood puts dangerous pressure on the brain, and the presence of the blood itself is like a huge bruise that irritates and damages normal brain tissue.

When an aneurysm bursts, it causes a sudden, severe headache, nausea, vomiting, and even unconsciousness. A neuro-surgeon must operate to remove the blood and to repair the broken blood vessel. Some people die when an aneurysm blows, but many survive. Unlike a torn balloon, a human blood vessel can often be repaired.

Stroke

Imagine that your grandfather has had a stroke. You go to the hospital with your parents to visit him, but he doesn't seem to recognize you. He can't move his right arm to feed himself. He can't use his right leg to walk. Sometimes he makes sounds, but you can't understand any words. You take his right hand, but it feels limp and he doesn't even know that you're holding it.

What happened? Something went terribly wrong inside your grandfather's brain. In eight out of ten strokes, a blood clot or air bubble (embolus) suddenly blocks an artery in the brain. When that happens, oxygen-rich blood can't reach the part of the brain that the blocked artery normally nourishes. Without oxygen, brain cells are injured almost immediately.

In two out of ten strokes, an artery or vein inside the brain actually bursts (much like an aneurysm). This floods the delicate brain tissue with blood—creating a hemorrhage. The brain suffers in two ways with a hemorrhage. Part of the brain doesn't get enough oxygen, and the presence of blood in brain cells is very damaging. This kind of stroke is usually worse than one caused by an embolism. People who suffer this type of stroke often have very high blood pressure.

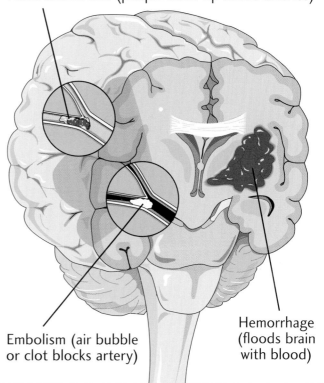

3 COMMON CAUSES OF STROKE

Atheroschlerosis (plaque build-up inside arteries)

Embolism (air bubble or clot blocks artery)

Hemorrhage (floods brain with blood)

What caused your grandfather's stroke? Chances are good that it was atherosclerosis. Atherosclerosis is a condition in which a fatty substance called plaque builds up along the walls of arteries. As it builds, the space inside the arteries narrows, so less blood flows through them. Pieces of plaque can break off and float in the bloodstream until they lodge in an artery narrowed by atherosclerosis.

Often, the plaque comes from the big carotid arteries, which are located on each side of the neck. An irregular heartbeat might cause a small blood clot to release from the heart and then lodge in an artery in the brain. Other things that can contribute to a stroke are diabetes, high cholesterol, and cigarette smoking.

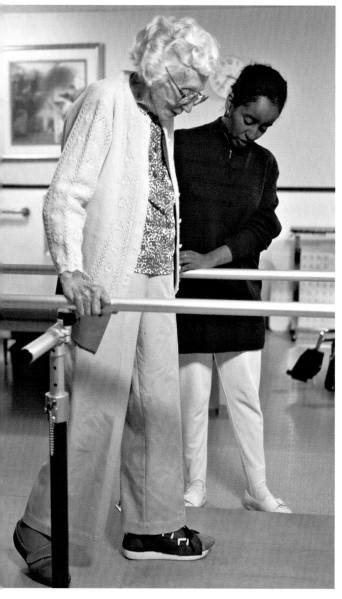

Physical therapy is often a part of recovering from a stroke.

The symptoms of a stroke depend on which arteries in the brain are affected. If you are ever with a person who suddenly develops any of the following symptoms, call 911 right away:

• Numbness or weakness of face, arm, or leg—usually on one side of the body.

• Confusion, trouble talking or understanding words.

• Trouble seeing in one or both eyes.

• Problems with walking, dizziness, or loss of balance.

• Sudden severe headache without any known reason.

The faster a person gets to the hospital during or after a stroke, the better the chance of a good recovery. In an emergency room, doctors can give intravenous medications that dissolve blood clots in the brain. When the blood clot is dissolved, the flow of oxygen-rich blood resumes and saves some of the injured brain cells.

About 300,000 people in the United States have strokes each year. About 25 percent of those people die. Half of the survivors are left with serious disabilities, such as weakness or paralysis on one side of the body.

The Right Brain-Left Brain Puzzle

The doctor tells your parents that your grandfather had a stroke of the middle cerebral artery in the left side of his brain. How can that be? It's his right arm and right leg that don't work correctly.

The left side of your brain actually controls movements on the right side of your body. If your grandfather had a stroke in the right side of his brain, it would affect movement of the left side of his body.

But what about his speech? Let's say your grandfather is right-handed. Speech control is in the left side of the brain for nearly all right-handed people. So damage to the left side of your grandfather's brain also causes problems with his speech.

Left-handed people are a little different. About 70 percent of them also have the speech center in the left side of the brain. Of the other 30 percent, some have the speech center in the right side of the brain, and some have it divided between left and right.

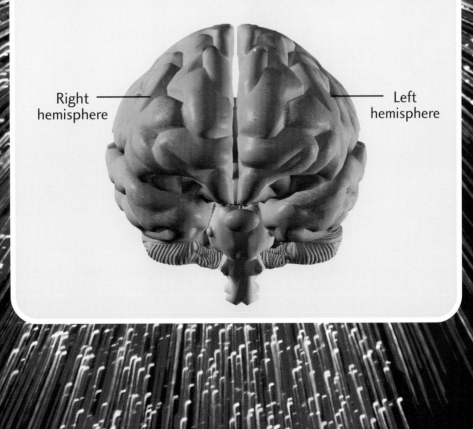

Right hemisphere ——— ——— Left hemisphere

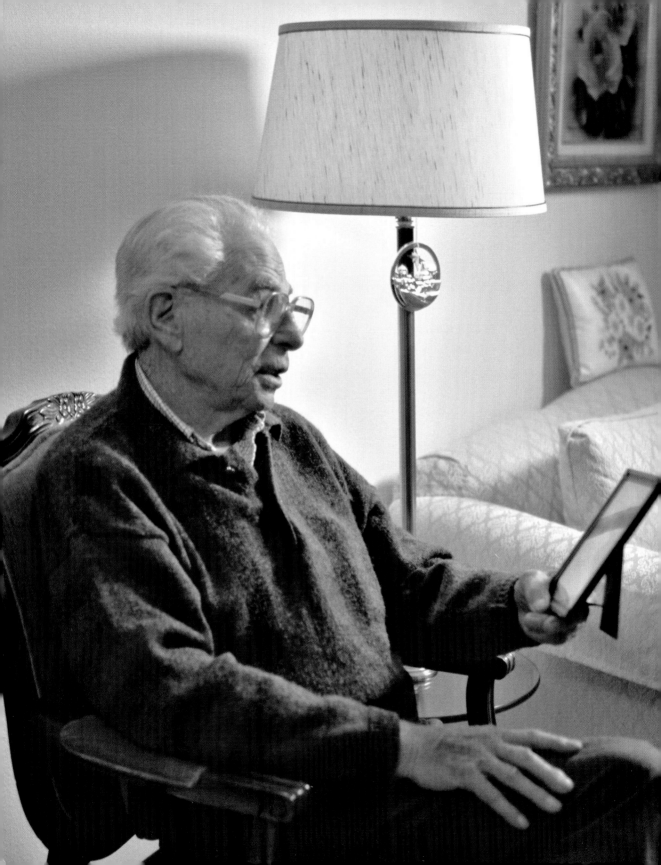

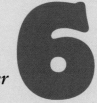

Degenerative Diseases

Multiple Sclerosis, Parkinson's Disease, and Alzheimer's Disease

Imagine for a moment what it would be like to find out you have a disease that can't be cured—a disease that will keep getting worse, no matter what you do. As the disease gets worse, your muscles stop working properly. You slowly lose the ability to speak. Your mind deteriorates. These are the effects of degenerative brain diseases.

The three major disorders covered in this chapter are quite different from each other, but they're grouped together because they each worsen over time. They differ in when they strike people and the symptoms they cause. But they have two things in common—they can't be cured yet, and they never go away.

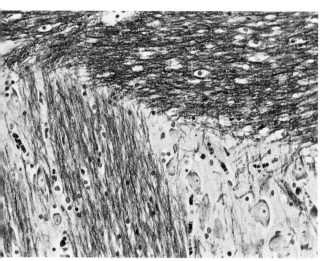

This microphotograph shows the structure of myelin.

Multiple Sclerosis

Picture a busy highway where traffic is whizzing along. Suddenly, cars reach a stretch where chunks of asphalt have been torn from the pavement. Most cars are forced to stop, but a few creep by in the side lane. This is how multiple sclerosis (MS) affects the central nervous system. Some nerve impulses reach their intended destination—an eye, an arm or leg, but many are delayed or entirely blocked.

About 350,000 people in the United States have MS. The disease tends to strike people early in life. Symptoms often appear for the first time between the ages of 20 and 40, and more women than men get it. Scientists are still trying to figure out the exact cause of MS. Many believe a combination of factors—genetics, viruses, the environment, and problems of the immune system—are to blame.

Myelin is a fatty substance that coats the axons of neurons in the brain and spinal cord. It is somewhat like the insulation that covers electrical wires. Myelin protects nerves and ensures that electrochemical messages travel rapidly and smoothly. With MS, the myelin becomes damaged and no longer allows nerves to transmit impulses efficiently. The symptoms of MS depend on the location of the myelin-damaged nerves. Common symptoms include swelling of the optic nerve, which can result in partial

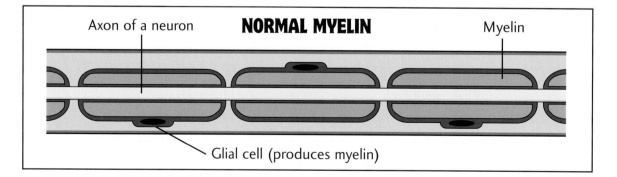

NORMAL MYELIN

Axon of a neuron

Myelin

Glial cell (produces myelin)

blindness, and extreme fatigue and weakness. Abnormal sensations—prickles or numbness in the arms and legs—may be another symptom of MS. In severe cases, MS may cause spastic muscles, tremors, poor bladder control, and problems with thinking, concentration, and memory.

It is tricky to diagnose MS, because symptoms can come and go, and vary with each person. An MRI scan can show damaged myelin in the brain and spinal cord. Much research continues to be done into the causes of MS and its treatments.

Scientists at Cornell University Medical College in New York have located the cells in the brain that grow into the myelin-making cells called oligodendrocytes. In the future, these cells may be implanted into the brains of people with MS. They may help MS sufferers to grow new myelin along damaged nerves.

In Michigan, researchers at the Mayo Clinic have grown new myelin in mice that have a disease similar to MS. This same procedure may be tested in humans in the near future. Doctors at the University of Southern California are testing a vaccine that specifically kills the immune cells that attack myelin.

Parkinson's Disease

Before actor Michael J. Fox publicly announced that he suffers from Parkinson's disease, most people thought it was only a disease of the elderly. While the average age of onset is 60, researchers are noting an increase in the number of young people developing Parkinson's disease. Up to 10 percent of

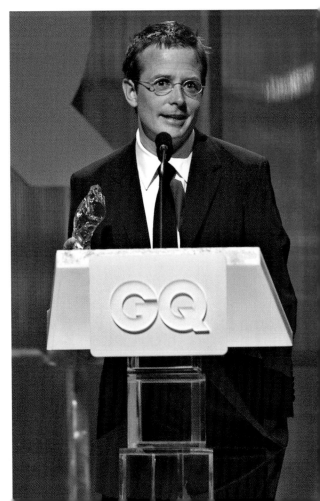

Actor Michael J. Fox has become an active spokesperson for Parkinson's sufferers.

Parkinson's cases are now diagnosed in people under 40. About half a million Americans have the disease, and 50,000 more are diagnosed with it every year.

Parkinson's disease is caused by the destruction of nerve cells in an area of the brain called the substantia nigra. These important cells produce the neurotransmitter dopamine, which is responsible for transmitting nerve impulses that coordinate movement. When the brain doesn't have enough dopamine, a person has problems with moving, walking, and balance.

Scientists know what happens in the brain with Parkinson's disease, but they don't know why it happens. Like multiple sclerosis, Parkinson's may be caused by a combination of factors. Some researchers believe the disease is linked to environmental toxins, such as pesticides and certain drugs. Others believe things called free radicals (unstable and potentially damaging molecules in the body) are the cause. A great number also recognize that genetics and aging are other important factors.

The early symptoms of Parkinson's disease develop gradually. People can feel shaky and tired. Then they might have trouble getting out of a chair. Eventually, handwriting may become cramped and spidery as tremors and shaking take hold. Family members may also notice a sudden lack of facial expression.

Most people finally seek medical help when their hands start shaking. The most classic symptoms of Parkinson's disease are

- **Tremor.** This shaking usually begins in one hand, with the thumb and forefinger doing a movement called "pill rolling." The tremor gets worse when the hand is resting, and decreases when the person reaches for something.
- **Rigidity.** The brain communicates poorly with muscles, which causes a state of constant muscular tension. A normal brain coordinates the balance of contraction and relaxation present with normal muscle movement. When someone tries to move the arm of a person with Parkinson's, it moves with short, jerky motions.

- **Slow movements.** People with Parkinson's lose the ability to perform routine activities, such as eating and dressing. Eating breakfast can take an hour instead of 10 minutes.
- **Unstable balance.** Poor balance and coordination are another hallmark of advanced Parkinson's disease. Sufferers tend to lean forward or backward in an attempt to stand upright. As the disease progresses, the body may "freeze" in place or topple over.

A medication called levodopa (L-dopa) is the standard treatment for Parkinson's disease. Nerve cells use this chemical to make dopamine and replenish the brain's supply. L-dopa delays the onset of Parkinson's disabling symptoms for many people, but it becomes less effective over time and has serious side effects. Newer medications and research are improving treatments every day. Many researchers believe that a cure for Parkinson's disease—as well as other similar brain disorders—is within our reach during the next 10 years.

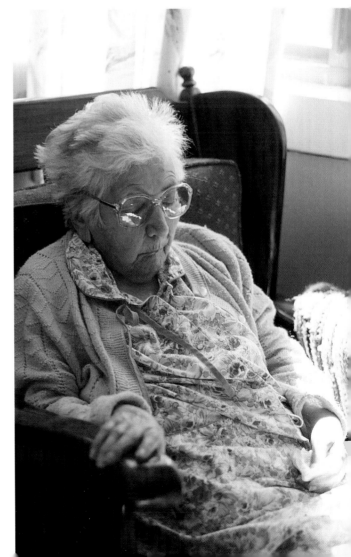

Alzheimer's is a disease most often brought on by old age.

Alzheimer's Disease

While Alzheimer's disease occasionally strikes people as young as 30, it is mainly considered a disease of old age. About 4 million Americans have it. Alzheimer's affects 1 in 10 people over 65 and nearly half of those over 85. As the huge wave of baby boomers ages, the number of Alzheimer's patients is expected to increase dramatically.

The Fight Against Alzheimer's

In 1994, millions of people were saddened when former President Ronald Reagan announced in a handwritten letter that he was suffering from Alzheimer's disease. He ended the letter by saying, "I now begin the journey that will lead me into the sunset of my life."

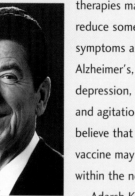
Ronald Reagan

President Reagan's wife, Nancy, became his full-time caretaker. His daughter, Maureen Reagan, began a crusade against Alzheimer's with the goal of raising $1 billion for research. Today, the U.S. government and the Alzheimer's Association lead the way in this research. Factors such as genetics, the role of estrogen in the brain, deficiencies of neurotransmitters, and problems in brain cell communication are all primary areas of study.

The Food and Drug Administration has approved three drugs that may temporarily delay the progression of the disease. Other medications and therapies may help to reduce some of the symptoms associated with Alzheimer's, such as depression, sleeplessness, and agitation. Scientists believe that a preventive vaccine may be developed within the next 10 years.

Adarsh Kumar, Ph.D., associate professor of psychiatry and behavioral sciences at the University of Miami, found that music therapy helped Alzheimer's patients sleep better. The music increased the level of melatonin, one of the brain's neurotransmitters.

Frederick Tims, Ph.D., is a music therapist at Michigan State University in East Lansing. He held music therapy sessions for Alzheimer's patients. Dr. Tims reported the participants were learning and singing songs, and were engaging in social interactions—unusual activities for Alzheimer's patients.

Could it be that music will have a place in the future as a regularly prescribed treatment for Alzheimer's?

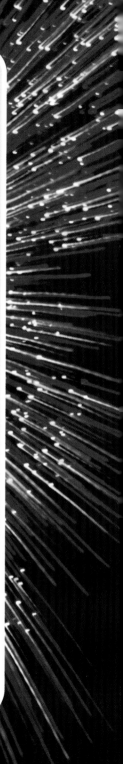

The onset of Alzheimer's is subtle, and its symptoms are often mistaken for those of normal aging. Dementia is a general term for a group of symptoms that can apply to Alzheimer's patients, though other forms of dementia besides Alzheimer's exist. Symptoms of dementia include a gradual loss of memory, especially for recent events; an inability to learn new information; and an increasing sense of anxiety, depression, and confusion. Other symptoms may include a growing tendency to misplace objects, and disorientation in familiar surroundings. Social skills slowly begin to break down, as do judgment and personality.

Like so many other neurological disorders, the exact cause of Alzheimer's disease is unclear. The brains of most patients show a characteristic pattern of plaques and tangles inside. The plaques are formed from dead and dying brain cells. The tangles are clumps of twisted protein fragments inside destroyed nerve cells.

After eliminating possibly treatable causes of dementia, a doctor will make a tentative diagnosis of Alzheimer's. But the disease cannot be diagnosed for certain until after a patient's death. If plaques and tangles are found in the brain tissue at autopsy, this confirms the presence of Alzheimer's disease.

Currently, there is no cure for Alzheimer's disease, nor any way to significantly slow its progression. Medications may relieve some symptoms, but ultimately, the disease is fatal in six to ten years.

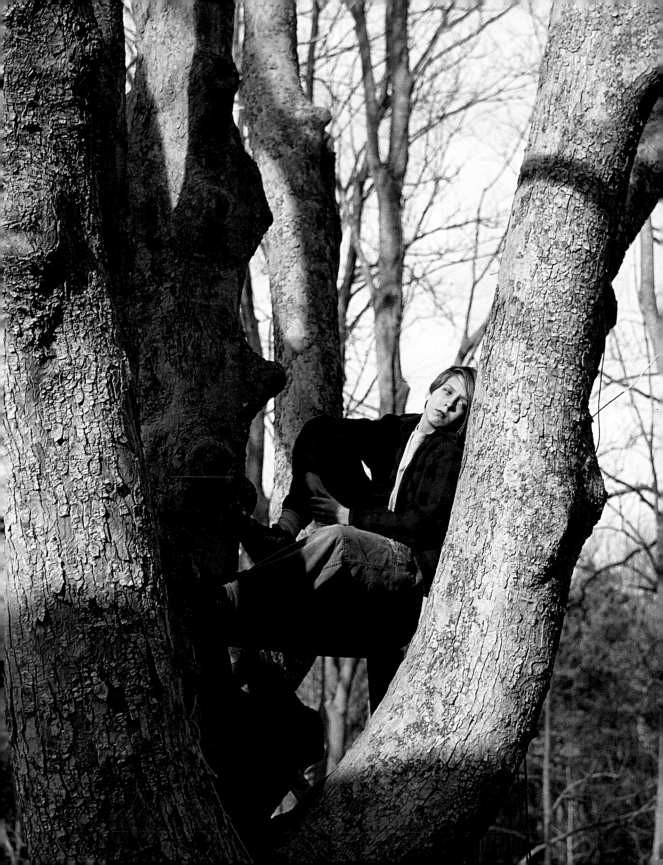

Chapter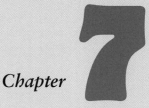

Brain and Mind

Tourette Syndrome, Autism, and Mental Illness

What would happen if the chemicals in your brain were mixed up, or some nerve cells didn't work properly? Your foot might twitch uncontrollably and the person next to you might get angry from being kicked. You might not be interested in talking to anyone; instead you might spend hours watching your fingers. Or, you could even hear voices that aren't real, telling you things that aren't true.

Some neurological disorders were once believed to be mental problems that needed to be treated by a psychiatrist. Scientists now know that Tourette syndrome, autism, and several mental illnesses may be largely due to chemical imbalances or structural abnormalities in the brain.

Tourette Syndrome

The boy sitting next to you starts twitching or grunting for no reason. He taps his foot and blinks all the time. He coughs and sniffs. At inappropriate times, he blurts out words or phrases. This boy might have Tourette syndrome. Tourette syndrome is a neurological disorder characterized by frequent involuntary movements and vocal sounds called tics. About 100,000 Americans have Tourette, and three times as many males have it as females. The disease is usually first noticed in childhood or adolescence, between the ages of 2 and 15.

Research suggests that an abnormal gene causes problems in how the brain uses the neurotransmitters dopamine and serotonin. Neurotransmitters are chemicals that travel across the microscopically small spaces (synapses) between nerve cells in the brain. If these chemicals don't work properly, nerve impulses are not conducted properly.

While no two Tourette syndrome patients are the same, all will display both motor (movement) and vocal tics. Some common motor tics are repeated blinking, facial grimaces, and foot tapping. Vocal tics include shouts, grunts, or repeating other people's words. The tics often decrease during sleep, or when concentrating on an activity. Every person with Tourette syndrome has his or her own pattern of tics, which can change over time. Although Tourette does not affect intelligence, some people with it have learning disabilities, attention problems, or compulsive behavior.

Serotonin molecule

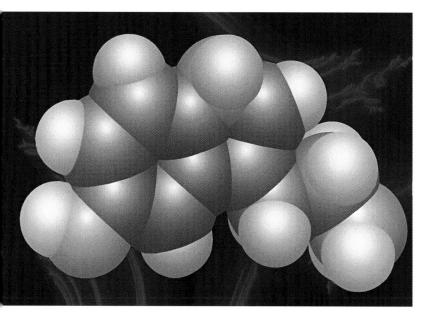

Autism

Most babies and toddlers are active, babbling, giggling, curious about the world around them. They love to be with people and to play with other kids. It is very different for children with autism. Autism is a disorder in which certain parts of the brain—the amygdala, hippocampus, and cerebellum, among others—fail to develop normally before birth. Abnormal development means brain neurons are unusually small and nerve fibers are stunted, which leads to problems with normal neural communication.

Scientists think a combination of genetic defects, viruses, and environmental chemicals can cause the abnormal brain development, but no one has identified the cause for certain.

Autism affects as many as one in 500 children in the United States—it strikes boys four times more often than girls. Autism is often diagnosed in infancy when a baby fails to achieve usual age-specific behaviors. Some children seem normal at first, but between 18 and 36 months, they lose skills and abilities. As this happens, they may develop impaired social interaction: failure to develop friends; inability to share with others; avoidance of eye contact and touch; and a failure to display normal emotions.

Autism is a disorder that may be caused by abnormal development of nerve fibers in the brain before birth.

Other classic indications of autism include faulty communication (delayed or absent language development; inability to start or maintain conversations with others; lack of normal childhood play) and other abnormal behavior (preoccupation with one activity; repetitive movements like flapping hands, rocking body, or head banging).

There's no blood test or X-ray to diagnose autism. If a doctor suspects the problem, a child will be sent to a specialist to confirm the diagnosis. Some people with autism are relatively high functioning, with intact speech and intelligence. Others are profoundly affected, mute, retarded, and closed off to the world.

Mental Illness

SCHIZOPHRENIA

Wouldn't it be frightening to hear voices you knew weren't really there? What if you were not able to tell reality from fantasy? These are common symptoms of schizophrenia. This disabling disease affects more than 2 million Americans—about 1 percent of the entire population. It usually strikes in adolescence or early adulthood and can make otherwise healthy, young people unable to function or interact with others. Schizophrenia is terrifying to the person who has it, and overwhelming to family and friends. What makes the devastating symptoms even more terrifying is that they appear suddenly. The most common symptoms of schizophrenia include hallucinations (seeing things and hearing voices that aren't real), and paranoia (belief that people are against you). Schizophrenics also commonly believe that others can hear their thoughts or control their actions. In addition, a schizophrenic suffers from disordered thinking, loss of concentration, and an inability to sort out what's real.

While schizophrenia is classified as a mental illness, new research suggests that it may be due to the complex interaction of several factors. Scientists discovered that people with schizophrenia have enlarged ventricles in the brain and a smaller hippocampus, which is important for learning and memory. The disease is also commonly hereditary—it runs in families, although a specific genetic defect hasn't yet been identified.

Other research suggests that schizophrenics have an imbalance of neurotransmitters in their brains. Studies of brain tissue also show microscopic abnormalities of nerve cells. Schizophrenia

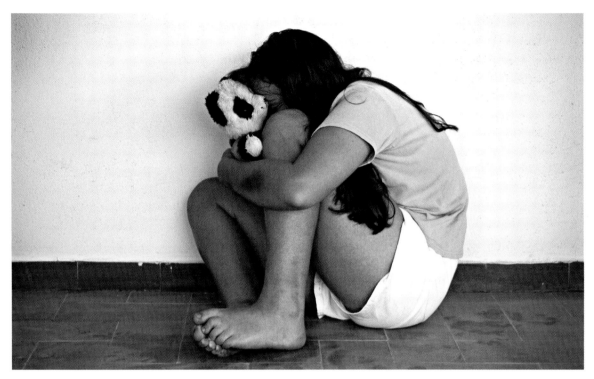

may be a developmental disorder that results from neurons forming incorrect connections before birth. These neurological errors lie dormant until triggered by normal changes in the brain during adolescence.

Medications can dramatically improve the life of schizophrenic patients. Even with medications, however, schizophrenics often suffer from problems in forming personal relationships, or holding down jobs. Schizophrenics are seldom violent, but their "bizarre" behavior sometimes frightens other people. Only one in five people with schizophrenia is ever considered "cured."

Many severe mental illnesses—such as schizophrenia—cause sufferers to withdraw and become disconnected from the people around them.

Obsessive-Compulsive Disorder

Did you ever hear the common saying, "Step on a crack, break your mother's back?" If you truly believed that, and spent all your time thinking about it while you walked, you would know a little of what it is like to have an obsessive-compulsive disorder (OCD). People with OCD suffer from recurrent unwanted

Autism—Past and Future

The Autistic Professor

Temple Grandin's symptoms began at 6 months old. She refused to be held, and was hypersensitive to sound, smell, and touch. She screamed and threw things. Sometimes she 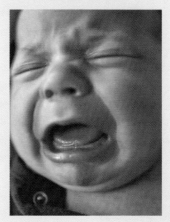 withdrew completely and watched her hands for hours at a time.

A doctor advised Temple's mother to put her in an institution, but she refused. Instead, she looked for a special school for her daughter. With intensive training, Temple later entered the regular school system. She completed high school and on went to college, where she earned a degree in animal science. Temple is a college professor who also writes and speaks about autism.

Temple has a unique ability to think in whole pictures. She can completely design a project or building in her mind, then draw it perfectly the first time. Despite these achievements, she doesn't understand most human emotions. Temple often describes herself as feeling like "an anthropologist on Mars."

Can Looking at Pictures Cure Autism?

At Yale University, Dr. Robert Schultz and colleagues have discovered when children with autism look at faces, they show a different pattern of brain activity than people without autism. Normal infants focus on faces and become experts at processing them in an area of the brain called the fusiform gyrus. Autistic children prefer looking at objects rather than faces. Facial expressions are meaningless to them.

A possible future treatment for autism could include getting infants and children who have been diagnosed with autism to spend time gazing at faces. This may help develop defective areas of the brain and improve social interaction.

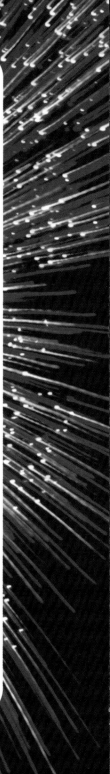

thoughts and the need to perform rituals over and over again. Common rituals include repeated hand washing, counting, or cleaning things. Performing these rituals provides only temporary relief from the excessively repetitive thoughts flooding through the OCD mind. Not performing these rituals only increases an already high level of anxiety.

There's growing evidence that OCD is due to abnormal functioning of circuits in the brain. Many researchers think OCD probably involves a part of the brain called the striatum. Special scans can show this abnormal brain structure. OCD is best treated through a combination of medications and behavioral therapy.

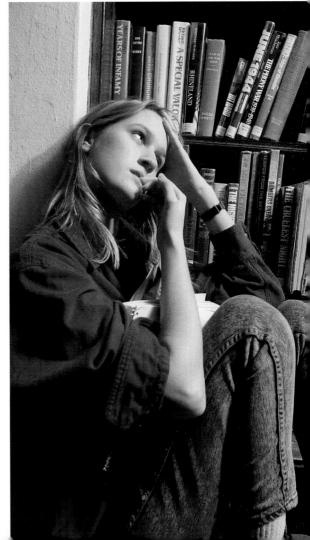

People with OCD are flooded with thoughts, anxiety, and a need to perform rituals.

BIPOLAR DISORDER

Bipolar disorder is also known as manic-depressive illness, and about 1 percent of the population has it. People with this disorder display extreme behavior that goes from deep depression to hyperactive, uncontrollable activity and racing thoughts.

Abnormalities in brain chemistry, and in the structure and activity of certain brain circuits, are responsible for the rapid shifts in mood and energy that characterize bipolar disorder. Without treatment, up to 20 percent of people with severe, untreated bipolar disorder will commit suicide. Medications and psychotherapy can help relieve symptoms for many people.

DEPRESSION

Everyone gets blue when things go wrong, and most people have been a little depressed at some time in their lives.

Living with Tourette Syndrome

In 1885, French neurologist Gilles de la Tourette first described the syndrome that now bears his name. In the next few years, hundreds of cases were discovered, each being different from one another. Some patients with severe cases of TS were described as being possessed. By the turn of the century, however, most doctors believed there was no such disorder.

It wasn't until the 1970s, when Dr. Oliver Sacks, a well-known British neurologist, began to notice "Touretters," as he called them, on the streets of New York City. He told himself that, "Tourette Syndrome must be very common, but is not recognized as such; once recognized, it's easily and frequently seen."

Michael is an 8th grader in California who knows all about TS; he's had it since the 3rd grade. Here's what he has to say about it:

"It's hard to describe what tics feel like. One tic I get is having to jump and hit my ankles together. Most of the time I just do it. But if I try to stop it, I get this feeling where the tic is wanting to happen, and it grinds on my nerves until I let the tic do its thing. So I can stop tics, but only for a while, because the feeling I get from holding them in drives me crazy. Probably the hardest thing about TS is what I call the "blinkies," when I can't stop blinking and can't concentrate."

The National Institute of Neurological Disorders and Stroke sponsors research on TS, and awards grants to major medical institutions across the country. Recent research has shown that TS is an inherited genetic disorder that causes different symptoms in each patient. Scientists are also studying brain activity and structure, neurotransmitters, and the environment, to determine what role these factors have in the development of TS.

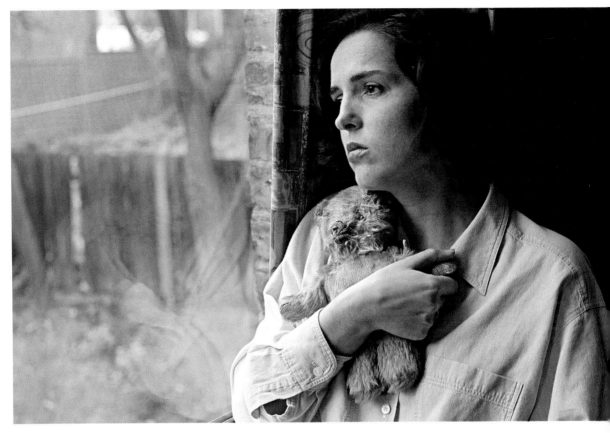

Severe and lasting depression, however, is very different, and it affects nearly 10 percent of the population. In fact, major depression is the leading cause of disability in the United States. Like other mental illnesses, major depression is proving to be both a psychiatric and a medical illness. Brain scans are showing that during depression, some of the brain circuits responsible for daily activities fail to function properly. It appears that the proper regulation of critical neurotransmitters, such as norepinephrine and serotonin, is impaired.

Organizations such as the National Institute of Mental Health continue to research the genetic and physiological causes of mental illness. Better therapies and medications are being developed to improve the lives of those suffering from many kinds of mental illnesses.

Recent studies show that during depression some of the brain's circuits do not function properly and the regulation of certain neurotransmitters is disrupted.

Glossary

Alzheimer's disease Decline of memory, thinking, intellect and function caused by irreversible changes in the brain.

Aneurysm A weakness in the wall of an artery or vein in the brain that may burst, sending a flood of blood into brain tissue.

Antibodies Substances produced by the body's immune system to help fight off invading organisms.

Atherosclerosis Deposits of fatty materials on the inside of arteries that can cause strokes and heart attacks.

Aura Unusual neurological symptoms (like flashing lights or numbness) that some people have before seizures or migraine headaches.

Autism A brain disorder in which a child fails to develop social and communication skills, and instead withdraws from people and normal activities.

Axon The part of a neuron that carries impulses away from the cell body.

Bell's palsy A paralysis of the facial nerve that leaves one side of the face sagging. Can be due to infections of the central nervous system.

Benign A tumor or condition that is probably not life-threatening.

Central nervous system (CNS) The brain, spinal cord, and cranial nerves.

Cerebral palsy (CP) A disorder caused by damage to parts of the brain that control muscle movements.

Cerebrospinal fluid (CSF) Fluid produced in the ventricles of the brain that helps to protect the brain and spinal cord.

Chemotherapy Strong medications used to treat cancer.

Coma A deep state of unconsciousness from which a patient cannot be aroused.

Contracture The abnormal shortening of a muscle, making it difficult to stretch it. Contractures are common in patients with cerebral palsy.

Cranial nerves The set of 12 nerves that control movement and sensation of the eyes, ears, nose, face, and tongue.

CT scan Computerized tomography—a medical examination in which computers make images of thin slices of the body, often used to diagnose neurological problems.

Degenerative disease A description of a disease like Parkinson's or Alzheimer's disease, in which patients steadily get worse over time.

Dementia A general loss of brain functions like memory, speech, and thinking.

Dendrite Part of neurons that receive impulses from other neurons.

Electroencephalogram (EEG) A recording of the electrical activity of the brain.

Embolus A blood clot or other material that suddenly blocks blood flow in an artery.

Encephalitis An infection of the brain, most often by a virus or bacterium.

Epilepsy An abnormality of the brain's transmission of electrical charges; a seizure disorder.

Hemorrhage The sudden escape of blood from a ruptured artery or vein; uncontrolled bleeding.

Hydrocephalus A buildup of cerebrospinal fluid in the brain leading to a dangerous increase in pressure.

Inflammation A swelling of injured tissues.

Laser Special light waves that can be used instead of scalpels for some kinds of surgeries.

Lyme disease A bacterial disease carried by ticks that can affect the central nervous system and other parts of the body.

Malignant A term used to refer to dangerously aggressive cancers that grow and spread rapidly.

Meninges The three layers of tissue-thin membranes that cover and protect the brain and spinal cord.

Meningitis An infection and inflammation of the meninges.

Migraine Severe disabling headache, thought to be caused by dilation and constriction of blood vessels in the brain.

MRI scan Magnetic resonance imaging—a special medical examination in which a patient is placed in a machine with a strong magnetic field. The test produces excellent images of the brain and other parts of the body.

Multiple sclerosis (MS) A disease in which the myelin that covers nerves is destroyed, impeding the transmission of nerve impulses throughout the body.

Myelin The fatty substance that covers the axons of neurons to help nerve impulses travel rapidly and smoothly.

Neurology The study of the nervous system.

Neuron The specialized cell of the nervous system composed of the cell body, dendrites, and axons. Neurons transmit electrical and chemical information to and from each other.

Neurotransmitter A chemical substance like dopamine and serotonin that travels between neurons to stimulate or inhibit them.

Nociceptors Special pain-sensitive neurons that let our bodies know when something hurts us.

Parkinson's disease A degenerative disease caused by the destruction of nerve cells in the brain that produce the neurotransmitter dopamine.

Photophobia An abnormal sensitivity to light.

Prostaglandin A group of natural chemicals in the body that perform many functions, one of which results in stimulating nociceptors to feel pain.

Radiation therapy The treatment of disease (usually cancer) by high-energy X-rays or gamma rays.

Schizophrenia A form of mental illness that may be caused partially by chemical imbalances in the brain. It results in people seeing, hearing, and believing things that aren't true, and inability to distinguish reality from fantasy.

Spinal tap A procedure that a doctor performs to take a sample of cerebrospinal fluid. A needle is inserted into the spine between the vertebrae and fluid is withdrawn.

Stroke A condition in which blood flow to the brain is interrupted by either a clot or a hemorrhage, causing serious damage to brain tissue.

Substantia nigra A group of cells in the brain that makes dopamine; the part of the brain damaged by Parkinson's disease.

Tic A rapid, involuntary, repetitive movement that occurs in patients with Tourette Syndrome.

Tourette Syndrome An inherited neurological disorder characterized by vocal and motor tics and some compulsive behaviors.

Ventricles Small chambers or cavities in the brain where cerebrospinal fluid is formed.

For More Information

BOOKS

Carson, Mary Kay. *Epilepsy*. Springfield, NJ: Enslow, 1998.

Gold, Susan Dudley. *Alzheimer's Disease*. Springfield, NJ: Enslow, Inc., 2000.

Gold, Susan Dudley. *Bipolar Disorder and Depression*. Springfield, NJ: Enslow, 2000.

Peacock, Judith. *Cerebral Palsy*. Mankato, MN: Capstone Press, 1999.

Peacock, Judith. *Epilepsy*. Mankato, MN: Capstone Press, 1999.

Peacock, Judith. *Mental Health: Bipolar Disorder*. Mankato, MN: Capstone Press, 2000.

Rosenberg, Marsha Sarah. *Everything You Need to Know When a Brother or Sister is Autistic*. New York: Rosen Publishing Group, 2000.

Sommers, Michael A. *Everything You Need to Know About Bipolar Disorder and Manic Depressive Illness*. New York: Rosen Publishing Group, 2000.

Susman, Edward. *Multiple Sclerosis*. Springfield, NJ: Enslow, 1999.

VanderHook, Sue. *Parkinson's Disease*. Mankato, MN: Smart Apple Media, 2000.

Veggeberg, Scott. *Lyme Disease*. Springfield, NJ: Enslow, 1998.

WEB SITES

Alzheimer's Association: http://www.alz.org

American Headache Society: http://ahsnet.org

Brain Injury Association, USA: http://www.biausa.org

Centers for Disease Control: http://www.cdc.gov

Epilepsy Foundation: http://www.epilepsyfoundation.org

Lyme Disease Foundation: http://www.lyme.org

National Brain Tumor Foundation: http://www.braintumor.org

National Headache Foundation: www.headaches.org

National Institute of Neurological Disorders and Stroke: http://www.ninds.nih.gov

National Institute of Mental Health: http://www.nimh.nih.gov

National Safe Kids Campaign: http://www.safekids.org

Index